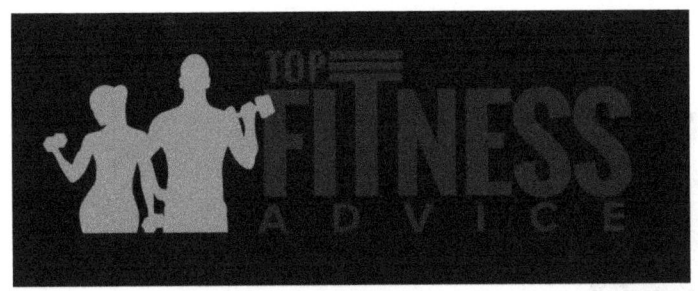

NO GYM WEIGHT LOSS

A Simple, Easy & PROVEN Guide to Build the Body of Your Dreams with NO GYM & NO WEIGHTS!

LINDA WESTWOOD

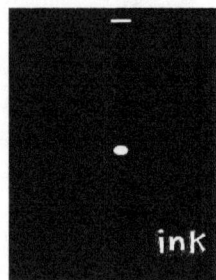

First published in 2017 by Venture Ink Publishing

Copyright © Top Fitness Advice 2019

All rights reserved.

No part of this book may be reproduced in any form without permission in writing from the author. No part of this publication may be reproduced or transmitted in any form or by any means, mechanic, electronic, photocopying, recording, by any storage or retrieval system, or transmitted by email without the permission in writing from the author and publisher.

Requests to the publisher for permission should be addressed to publishing@ventureink.co

For more information about the contents of this book or questions to the author, please contact Linda Westwood at linda@topfitnessadvice.com

Disclaimer

This book provides wellness management information in an informative and educational manner only, with information that is general in nature and that is not specific to you, the reader. The contents of this book are intended to assist you and other readers in your personal wellness efforts. Consult your physician regarding the applicability of any information provided in this book to you.

Nothing in this book should be construed as personal advice or diagnosis, and must not be used in this manner. The information provided about conditions is general in nature. This information does not cover all possible uses, actions, precautions, side-effects, or interactions of medicines, or medical procedures. The information in this book should not be considered as complete and does not cover all diseases, ailments, physical conditions, or their treatment.

You should consult with your physician before beginning any exercise, weight loss, or health care program. This book should not be used in place of a call or visit to a competent health-care professional. You should consult a health care professional before adopting any of the suggestions in this book or before drawing inferences from it.

Any decision regarding treatment and medication for your condition should be made with the advice and consultation of a qualified health care professional. If you have, or suspect you have, a health-care problem, then you should immediately contact a qualified health care professional for treatment.

No Warranties: The author and publisher don't guarantee or warrant the quality, accuracy, completeness, timeliness, appropriateness or suitability of the information in this book, or of any product or services referenced in this book.

The information in this book is provided on an "as is" basis and the author and publisher make no representations or warranties of any kind with respect to this information. This book may contain inaccuracies, typographical errors, or other errors.

Liability Disclaimer: The publisher, author, and other parties involved in the creation, production, provision of information, or delivery of this book specifically disclaim any responsibility, and shall not be held liable for any damages, claims, injuries, losses, liabilities, costs, or obligations including any direct, indirect, special, incidental, or consequences damages (collectively known as "Damages") whatsoever and howsoever caused, arising out of, or in connection with the use or misuse of the site and the information contained within it, whether such Damages arise in contract, tort, negligence, equity, statute law, or by way of other legal theory.

Table of Contents

Disclaimer	3
Who is this book for?	7
What will this book teach you?	9
Introduction	11
Chapter 1: Target Real Achievements but Build Slowly	17
Chapter 2: 10 Beginner Workouts	31
Chapter 3: 10 Intermediate Workouts	37
Chapter 4: 10 Advanced Workouts	43
Chapter 5: Morning Habits	51
Chapter 6: Afternoon Habits	63
Chapter 7: Evening Habits	73
Chapter 8: Tracking Your Progress	79
Conclusion	85
Final Words	89

Would you prefer to listen to my book, rather than read it?

Download the audiobook version for free!

If you go to the special link below and sign up to Audible as a new customer, you can get the audiobook version of my book completely free.

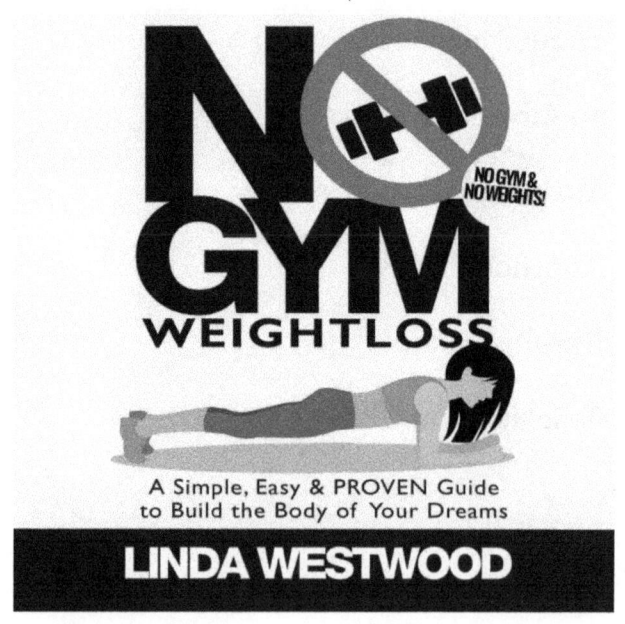

Go here to get your audiobook version for free:

TopFitnessAdvice.com/go/NoGym

Who is this book for?

Do you lack enthusiasm for sports or going to the gym?

Are you put off by the bother of it all and the sheer hard work involved?

Proven scientific research tells us that we need to keep active if we want to be healthy, but the guidelines are unrealistic for many of us. They tell us to walk so many thousand steps a day, do aerobic exercise three times a week, take up a sport or work out at the gym.

Some people seem to relish sports and gyms, and good for them.

But what about the rest of us, who either don't have the time, or lack the inclination?

What will this book teach you?

And as for following a diet plan – forget it!

Life's too short for cooking special 'calorie-counted' recipes, only to end up with an unsatisfying meal that you probably don't like and would never normally eat. It's just not sustainable long-term.

How can you avoid going back to your old eating habits the minute you stop following your diet plan?

In an ideal world, you would be able to eat all your usual favorite foods without worrying, and stay at a healthy weight. And you wouldn't have to spare some precious time for exercise, or go out of your way to do it.

It sounds impossible…

But wait, there might be a way!

I'm going to share with you my tips for living a fitter and healthier life, and you won't have to find any more time in your day to accomplish it. Nor will you have to eat any different foods that you don't like, or go without anything that you do like.

Does it sound too good to be true?

Well, it's worked for me.

Through a desire to be as healthy as I can be, without compromising my enjoyment of life, I have developed a simple method that anyone can use, even if you hate exercise and have no willpower to deny yourself the foods you like best.

Introduction

I have managed to lose over a stone in weight over the past two years and feel stronger and more energetic, using the techniques described below.

You too can lose weight whilst still eating what you enjoy, and be fitter without making time for exercising. It's not a quick fix, but the important thing is to make changes for life, so that the new and healthier you is here to stay!

Read on to discover the secrets of the easy 'half and double' eating plan, the principles of 'kitchen yoga' and other revelations that you may not have thought about before, but which could help you live a healthier life.

Change Your Mind

We all know how difficult it is to stick to a diet. And even if we do stick to one for a while, as soon as we go back to what we perceive as eating 'normally' the weight creeps back on. So, let's approach this in a different way.

It's not so much about what we choose to eat, but more about learning to respect the food on our plates, and to stop eating more than we really need.

Before you start to eat, take a moment to admire your plate of food and think how lucky you are to have it. Imagine how delicious it's going to be. Don't eat whilst doing something else at the same time, but give your food the attention it deserves.

Be mindful of the eating experience, noticing your enjoyment of each mouthful. Learn to relish and savor food, as one of the great pleasures of life that it is.

It may seem obvious, but make sure that you don't eat anything you don't really enjoy. Ask yourself if the enjoyment of what you're eating is enough to make the calorie intake worthwhile. This is probably the most important thing to be mindful of.

If you are trying to lose weight, never eat anything that you're not really enjoying, and don't continue to eat when you're full. Never add empty calories to your daily intake, without the benefit of enjoyment.

Of course, if you happen to dislike vegetables, they are an obvious exception to the rule of not eating anything you're not enjoying. You can and should increase your vegetable intake, as most vegetables have negligible calorie content and they are packed with vitamins.

As you cut down on the more calorific parts of your meals, you can fill up with a larger serving of vegetables. There is a vast range of different types of vegetables to explore, so try to seek out new varieties and relish the excitement of new tastes and textures.

The 'Half and Double' Eating Plan

You don't have to cut out any of your normal meals or snacks, or deny yourself any food that you love (no matter how 'unhealthy' it may be). The trick is just to make your meals and snacks smaller.

To make things really easy, you could just halve everything you would normally eat. Again, the only exception to this is vegetables (excluding potatoes) of which you can have as many as you like.

As an example of the concept, if you'd normally eat a bar of chocolate or a cake with your afternoon cup of tea, you can still have it – but cut it in half before you start, and save the other half for the next time you'd normally have this snack.

So, you don't have to change what you eat, but just eat less of it. You don't have to cook any special 'diet' recipes, or count calories. If you are consistent with halving everything, you will quickly see the pounds start to drop off.

Eating your normal meals and snacks, but less of them, is also something you can probably stick to, as it doesn't involve any drastic changes in diet. Over time, you will find that you get used to eating smaller portions, and it will become a way of life.

Now, you may think that you'll be left feeling hungry and unsatisfied after your half-size meals, but the second part of the plan goes a long way towards preventing that. Try to take smaller mouthfuls (half your usual size) and really savor what you're eating. Notice the different tastes and textures, and the enjoyment your food gives you.

Savor every mouthful for twice as long as you normally would. This is the 'double' part of the plan. With practice, you will get into the habit of chewing more thoroughly.

If you'd normally chew a mouthful 10 times, try to make it 20 instead. Enjoy every bit of flavor you can. This will not only help you to feel more satisfied with a smaller amount of food, but will also help with digestion. It will slow down your eating so that your body will register a satisfied feeling more quickly.

You won't master your new way of eating overnight, but with practice it will become second nature. You should find that you are eating less, eating more slowly and enjoying each meal or snack just as much, if not more, than before.

So, it's simple – halve every portion, double every chew!

Keeping Busy

Even if you are doing well with your new eating plan, of course there will be lapses and cravings.

It's hard to resist that extra snack between meals when the opportunity to have it is there. So, when you find yourself thinking about crisps, biscuits, or whatever your weakness may be, remove the opportunity to give in to the craving by doing something else to occupy your mind.

You could go for a walk, tidy a drawer, clean out the fridge, try on outfits, do any sort of housework – the possibilities are endless. In fact, you could start by writing out a list of jobs you want to get done around the house, and refer to this list whenever you need a distraction activity, to stop you thinking about snacking.

You will become much more productive, and what you achieve will be a bonus, over and above the satisfaction of resisting those snacks.

Mini-Snacks

Of course, it's not always possible to resist snacking, and we all need little treats now and again. A cup of tea becomes much more enjoyable if it's accompanied by a biscuit or cake, and since our aim is to enjoy life as much as possible whilst staying as healthy as we can, we shouldn't deny ourselves small indulgences – 'small' being the operative word.

You can still have your snacks, as long as you make them much smaller, and really appreciate and savor them. You could go even further than just halving your snacks - even just one square of chocolate or a mouthful of biscuit is enough to make a cup of tea taste better. Just a sweet taste in your mouth may be all you need to satisfy you, not a whole slice of cake!

Chapter 1

Target Real Achievements but Build Slowly

Motivation

The two hardest parts of losing weight are starting your plan and then sticking with it.

Hopefully if you're reading this it means you've got the motivation to start, but chances are if you're like how I used to be you get a week in and then give up on your regime.

The first thing we tackle is how to get motivation and sustain it. The habits in this book are self-reinforcing; once you start them, you're going to love and do them more because you enjoy them.

Exercise

Whilst diet plays an important part in weight loss, exercise is much more important when you're getting down to the final 12-16 pounds. Your puppy fat will not shift on diet alone. As a result, we dedicate the mid-section to the art of exercise.

If you hate the gym then don't worry; you're going to learn to exercise smart, not hard, and you never need to go to a gym if you don't want to.

Diet

This is not a diet book.

There is no list of miracle foods or specific food types you cannot eat.

Diet is a hard thing to change, it is a habit ingrained into us by repeating the same actions every day. I have no urge to tell you what you can and cannot eat.

However, with some small adjustments to your routine and by making some sensible choices, combined with your sky-high motivation from section one you will finish this book having made the sustainable changes you need to lose that excess. And you can keep eating take out.

There's no time to lose, so let's dive straight into our first step - motivation.

Motivation

A marathon starts with a single step

Start Small

Well done on getting this far!

That might sound stupid, but one of the best pieces of advice I've been given is this: if you're trying to do something but you really lack the motivation to do it, just take the smallest first step towards it. It can be the tiniest amount of work, but once you've started that journey it's a lot easier to motivate yourself to continue it.

For example: you want to train to run 5 kilometers. That might sound pretty daunting, so you put it off.

What is the smallest step on this journey you can make? Probably packing your gym bag to take to work. You're not committing to doing the run, there's no guarantee it will happen. You're simply packing your bag. You're not too lazy to pack a bag surely?

But now it's your lunch break and you have a bag of gym gear. Still feeling hesitant? Commit to walking to the changing room. You don't even need to go inside, you can get a coffee next door if you change your mind, just make the walk.

Now you're in the changing room, so you should probably change. You don't have to run, you could just walk around, but you should at least change. And so on and so forth.

You'll quickly find you're actually doing whatever it is you set out to do by breaking it down into a series of smaller, more manageable steps. You've decided you want to lose those final pounds and get down to the weight you've always wanted.

That's potentially a long and daunting journey, but you've started it just by reading this book. Be proud! You should be proud of all of your achievements.

Build up to your targets and goals slowly. If you don't want to do something, start by doing the minimum possible amount of work that gets you towards that target.

Action: Think about something you don't want to do. It could be work, health, personal. What's the smallest step towards that goal you can make? Do it. What's next? Do that as well. Keep going till you achieve the goal.

Often the problem lies not in knowing how to lose weight but simply lacking the motivation to do so; you need a kickstarter. The best way of doing this is using specific, quantifiable goals. You have to set yourself a challenging but achievable target that will make you get up off your couch and start achieving it.

Again, let's go back to 5km training from the previous example. Let's modify it slightly by saying we want to run 5km every day. You may think you are capable of this, but unless you're in terrible health then you should be able to slowly walk 5km.

Begin with this and walk the full distance. Do this 3 times and you will already be feeling fitter. Then start jogging for a little bit of it. Then jog more. Then jog it all. Building it up slowly you will quickly find that each time you're achieving something new and that the feeling of success is very addictive and will keep you motivated to keep doing it. It is self-sustaining.

This technique applies not just to exercise but dieting too, and other aspects of life. Maybe you drink 3 cans of cola a day (not unheard of!). Start by cutting down gradually, maybe dropping to 2 cans every other day, then every day. Then down to 1 can, continuing until you're completely off.

Action: Set yourself a clear goal, which you can build up to with incremental improvements. Agree how often you're going to do/not do that thing. Stick to it by any means necessary.

Here are some example goals for you to choose from:

- Run a distance, such as 5 or 10km
- Walk to work every day
- Go for a bike ride every day
- Stop drinking fizzy drinks
- Stop drinking coffee/tea
- Bring lunch from home every day
- Only check Facebook once a day
- Read for half an hour every day

Embarrass Yourself Into Shape

There are lots of things that motivate us. Sometimes it can be a partner or friends telling us we've put on some weight. Perhaps it's having to replace your favorite wardrobe items because you can no longer do the buttons up. More often than not it's just because you want to feel good about yourself.

We are a society that is unhealthily fixated on looks, in particularly weight and being unachievably thin thanks to the menace of photoshop. The title of this book contains the words "lose weight", which is in itself is a misnomer. The key here is to lose fat, or even more specifically to tone up. Muscle weighs more than fat, so in reality I'd be quite happy to put on weight if I'm replacing my fat with muscle.

But how can we make the high-pressure nature of modern society work in our favor?

I have found great success by making goals and targets public. Right now, if you fail in your goal of increased exercise and a trimmer figure, the only person you're letting down is yourself. Only you know you're attempting this thing. However, making your goals public by telling friends and family is guaranteed to increase your motivation and chances of success. Why?

Embarrassment if you fail!

If you tell someone you are going to achieve something and then fall through on that commitment you look bad. You look flakey. You look like you can't commit to things. We're all built to hate this sort of feeling. We are brought up wanting to be reliable individuals, to think that our friends can count on us. We can channel this feeling to our advantage.

My colleagues on the other hand are the people that see me the most. When you first start succeeding, it's your colleagues who will be the first to remark that you've lost weight or are looking good. Announce to them early, and bring it up a couple of times a week. They may get annoyed at you for constantly going on about it, but they'll ultimately be understanding.

It also increases the guilt factor; they're not going to let you chow down on a lunchtime pizza without questions. It also means they'll be more sympathetic when not joining in on team lunches or if you stay off the booze when on a team night out. As we'll discuss in the diet section there's no need for extreme dieting, but there are some situations you'll want to say no. Announcing publicly helps.

This idea has been taken to extreme with ideas like Stickk. You select your goal but then set monetary stakes; for example, you could commit to losing 5kg in 6 weeks. If you fail, you will then give money (say, $100) to either a friend, a charity, or an anti-charity (a charity you would hate to give money to). Stickk claim that you are 3 times more likely to achieve your goals when there is money on the line.

Something important to note: It is important you are at risk of losing money as opposed to getting the opportunity to earn it. "I will give my friend $100 if I lose" is a lot more powerful than "I will buy myself that $100 dress" as a motivation. This is known in economics as "Loss Aversion".

People prefer to avoid losses than to acquire gains. Think about it for a minute; if you lose $100 when walking home you will be disproportionately unhappy relative to the enjoyment gained from finding $100.

This can go even further with an element of competition.

One of my favorite examples of this I picked up from some close friends who were recently engaged. In the build-up to their wedding they both wanted to lose weight, and committed to this via competition. They each put the equivalent of about 10USD into a pot at the start of the week, and then at the end they have a weigh in; whoever has lost the most weight gets to keep the money.

Whilst being exceptionally motivational (no one wants to lose!) it also has the advantage of playing both sides of the loss aversion curve; if you win you both avoid loss and acquire gain.

Action: Tell your friends and family your goals up front. Get the people closest to support and pressure you a little. Think about signing up to a website or app to help track your goal, and maybe put some money in as a bigger incentive.

You Can't Fix What You Don't Measure: Quantified Self

You may have heard the term "quantified self" being mentioned in the press recently as it has developed something of a cult following. But what does it mean, and specifically, what does it mean for you?

One of my favorite definitions of QS is this: "Quantified self is an advanced way of collecting data about an individual's life using technological tools. This includes the inputs, states and mental and physical performance that's achieved as a result. This type of tracking is used for self-improvement".

The quantified self provides the battle ground for the latest war between the leading technology companies. The latest iPhone has a co-processor dedicated to health tracking and a dedicated application for tracking everything from steps and heart rate to what you've been eating.

The recent onslaught of watches from Samsung, Apple, Motorola and others have all had features such as step counters and heart rate monitors. Dedicated devices such as Fitbit, Jawbone Up and Nike Fuelband have been flying off the shelves globally.

As technology has advanced and become cheaper it has allowed this market to flourish, but why are these new tools and technologies so useful? Simply put, you cannot fix what you don't measure.

I find it very frustrating when people say they want to lose weight but they refuse to get onto scales and weigh themselves. You cannot know if you're losing weight without measuring your weight!

Using a mirror and seeing if you look like you've lost weight is a terrible idea. I can guarantee if you look in the mirror after you've eaten cake, you'll feel you've put on weight when in reality it's not true.

Things like step counters, running apps and electronic scales can accurately and objectively show us the progress we are making along our journey. This is the only true measure.

The quantified self-movement helps by reducing the effort it takes to record this information and to present trends back. The AppStore contains thousands of applications to help you get and stay in shape, with everything from calorie counting to training plans.

In this chapter, we are going to discuss the steps you can take which, with minimal effort, will see a big transformation in your health and body shape.

Discover Scientifically-Proven "Shortcuts" & "Hacks" to Lose Weight FASTER (With Very Little Effort)

For this month only, you can get Linda's best-selling & most popular book absolutely free – *Weight Loss Secrets You NEED to Know.*

Get Your FREE Copy Here:

TopFitnessAdvice.com/Bonus

Discover scientifically-proven tips to help you lose weight faster and easier than ever before. With this book, readers were able to improve their weight loss results and fitness levels. So, it's highly recommended that you get this book, especially while it's free!

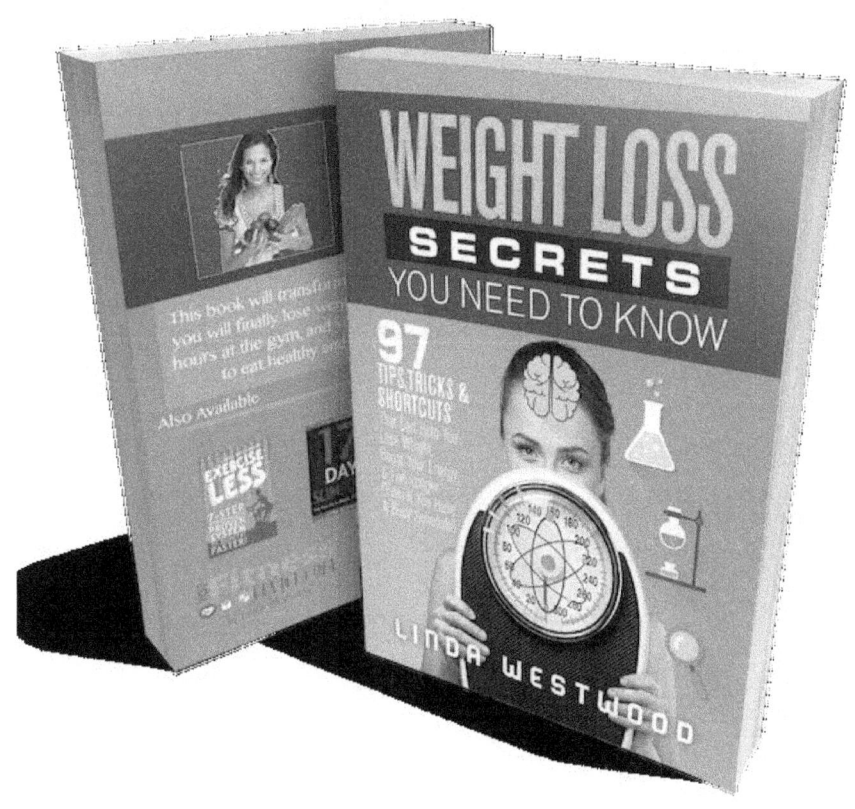

Get Your FREE Copy Here:

TopFitnessAdvice.com/Bonus

Chapter 2

10 Beginner Workouts

(1) 4 Sets of:

- 2:00 jump rope
- 30 seconds speed skipping
- 30 seconds plank
- 20 seconds mountain climbers

*Rest 20 seconds between exercises and 1:30 between sets.

NOTES: This workout will engage your core and test your skipping abilities. If you mess up during a timed skipping exercise in any of the workouts, try to get right back to the exercise as soon as you recover from your mistake.

(2) 4 X 25 reps of the following exercises:

- Single leg skip (right)
- Single leg skip (left)
- Ski Skips
- Crossovers
- Speed skipping

*No rest between exercises. Rest 2 minutes after each set.

NOTES: Try to transition between exercises as fast as possible. Don't waste any time!

(3) Complete 3 sets of the following:

- 100 jump rope
- 20 squat jumps
- 30 mountain climbers
- 40 jumping jacks
- 50 jump rope

*Rest 20 seconds between exercises and 2 minutes between sets.

(4) In 8 minutes, complete as many sets as you can:

- 30 speed skipping
- 5 burpees
- 15 speed skaters
- 10 squat jumps

*No designated rest at all during this workout. You're trying to see how many sets you can complete. Try to set a consistent pace and hold it for the entire 15 minutes.

Obviously, you will have to rest, but you should try to space out this rest time and minimize it as much as possible.

(5) 4 X 20 reps of the following exercises

- Pushups
- Crossovers
- Reverse Crunches
- Ski Skipping
- Seal Jacks

- Speed Skipping
- Mountain Climbers
- Boxing Jump Rope

*Rest 30 seconds between exercises and 2:30 minutes between sets.

NOTES: This workout will test your skipping ability by incorporating many different skipping techniques.

(6) Complete 2 sets of the following:

- 30 seconds jump rope
- 30 seconds plank
- 1:00 jump rope
- 1:00 plank
- 1:30 jump rope
- 1:30 plank
- 2:00 jump rope
- 2:00 plank

*No rest between exercises. Rest 3 minutes between sets.

NOTES: If you can't hold the plank for the specified time, simply take a short rest when you need to and then get right back into plank position as soon as you can.

(7) Perform each exercise for 45 seconds, rest for 30 seconds and then perform the same exercise for 30 seconds.

Once you do the exercise twice, rest for 1:30 and move down the list. Complete 1 set of the following:

- Speed skipping
- Burpees
- Wall sits
- Single leg skip (left)
- Single leg skip (right)
- Lunge walks
- Freestyle skipping

(8) In 20 minutes do as many jump ropes (or freestyle skipping) as you can.

Record the number in a workout journal so that you can do this work out again in the future and track your progress. You may find it difficult to keep count and it's not overly important that you do. The important thing is that you skip for 20 minutes straight. If you make mistakes resume skipping as soon as you can.

(9) 4 X 20 seconds of each exercise:

- Speed skipping
- Mountain climbers
- Ski skipping
- Push-ups
- Boxing jump rope
- Burpees

*Rest 20 seconds between exercises and 1 minute between sets.

NOTES: This workout is meant to be very intense. One set is complete once you do 20 seconds of each exercise. Push yourself as hard as you can during the 20-second pieces and try to do as many reps as you can.

(10) 6 X 30 reps of the following exercises:

- Boxing jump rope
- Single leg skip (right)
- Single leg skip (left)
- Ski Skips
- Crossovers
- Speed skipping
- Jumping jack skipping

*No rest between exercises. Rest 2 minutes after each set.

NOTES: Try to transition between exercises as fast as possible. Don't waste any time!

I hope that you are enjoying this book so far, and if you could spare 30 seconds, I would greatly appreciate you leaving a review on Amazon.com.

Chapter 3

10 Intermediate Workouts

(1) You have 15 minutes to complete all of the repetitions of the following exercises:

- 400 jump rope
- 30 burpees
- 60 push-ups
- 100 reverse crunches
- 50 lunge walks
- 100 double unders

*Rest as you need, but try to get it all done in 15 minutes.

NOTES: You don't have to go down the list as you would in a normal workout. For example, you could do 100 jump ropes, 10 lunge walks, 5 burpees, 20 push-ups, 30 reverse crunches, etc. Just make sure that you keep track of your repetitions. You could use a white board or a pen and paper.

(2) 2 X 10 minutes jump rope. Each 10 minutes is broken down as follows:

- 2:00 jump rope
- 1:00 speed skipping
- 30 seconds single leg skip (left leg)
- 30 seconds single leg skip (right leg)
- 1:00 ski skipping
- 1:00 boxing jump rope

- 30 seconds heel skipping
- 30 seconds crossovers
- 2:00 jumping jack skipping
- 1:00 double unders

*No rest during the 10 minutes. Rest 3 minutes between sets.

(3) Complete 2 sets of the following:

- 50 double unders, 50 jumping jacks
- 40 double unders, 40 seal jacks
- 30 double unders, 30 mountain climbers
- 20 double unders, 20 reverse crunches
- 10 double unders, 10 push ups
- 5 double unders, 5 burpees

*Rest 30 seconds between exercises (meaning that you rest only after the non-skipping exercises. For example, you would do 50 double unders, 50 jumping jacks and then rest for 30 seconds). Rest 3 minutes between sets

NOTES: Do double unders if possible. If you can't do double unders then do speed skipping for double the amount of jumps (Example: if you can't do 50 double unders then do 100 regular jumps as fast as you can).

(4) Complete one set of the following:

- 5:00 jump rope
- 50 seconds plank
- 4:00 freestyle skipping
- 40 seal jacks

- 3:00 freestyle skipping
- 30 lunge walks
- 2:00 speed skipping
- 20 squat jumps
- 1:00 speed skipping
- 10 push-ups

* Rest 30 seconds between exercises.

(5) Complete as many sets as possible in 10 minutes:

- 25 double unders
- 5 squat jumps
- 3 burpees

*Rest as needed but remember you want to see how many sets you can do. Try to minimize your rest time. For example, you could rest for 20 seconds only after you complete 3 sets.

NOTES: At first glance this workout may not seem like it will be too difficult, but don't fool yourself.

I purposely made the sets short so that you have to do a lot of them within the 10-minute period. This workout is sure to burn!

(6) Complete 4 sets of the following exercises:

- 2:00 freestyle skipping
- 1:30 plank
- 25 lunge walks
- 1:00 wall sit

- 15 squat jumps
- 20 double unders

*Rest 30 seconds between exercises and 2:00 between sets

NOTES: This workout is sure to push your legs to the limit!

(7) Complete 1 set of the following:

- 10 double unders, 1 push-up
- 9 double unders, 2 push-ups
- 8 double unders, 3 push-ups
- 7 double unders, 4 push-ups
- 6 double unders, 5 push-ups
- 5 double unders, 6 push-ups
- 4 double unders, 7 push-ups
- 3 double unders, 8 push-ups
- 2 double unders, 9 push-ups
- 1 double under, 10 push-ups
- REST FOR 2 MINUTES
- 1 double under, 10 push-ups
- 2 double unders, 9 push ups
- 3 double unders, 8 push-ups
- 4 double unders, 7 push-ups
- 5 double unders, 6 push-ups
- 6 double unders, 5 push-ups
- 7 double unders, 4 push-ups
- 8 double unders, 3 push-ups
- 9 double unders, 2 push-ups
- 10 double unders, 1 push-up

*Only rest at the halfway mark as instructed (for 2 minutes).

NOTES: This is a tough one, set a nice consistent pace and try to hold it the entire time.

(8) Perform 4 sets of the following:

- Max jump rope
- Max plank
- Max double unders

*Rest 2 minutes between exercises and 5 minutes between sets.

NOTES: Max means that you perform as many reps as you can before failure. In the case of plank, you simply hold the plank position for as long as you possibly can before quitting.

Once you fail, the exercise is over and the rest period begins. See how consistent you can be in your exercise reps. Push yourself to the limit on this workout!

(9) 6 Sets of the following:

- 1:00 speed skipping
- 10 squat jumps
- 30 seconds double unders
- 20 mountain climbers
- 1:00 speed skipping
- 30 seconds double unders

* Rest 30 seconds between exercises and 1:30 between sets.

(10) Perform 3 sets of the following:

- 150 jump rope
- 25 single leg skip (left)
- 25 single leg skip (right)
- 25 double unders
- 90 second plank
- 20 pushups 5 burpees
- 25 crossovers
- 25 jumping jack skipping
- 25 ski skipping
- 25 speed skipping

* Rest 20 seconds between exercises and 2 minutes between sets.

Chapter 4

10 Advanced Workouts

(1) 3 X 5 minutes unbroken jump rope.

*Rest 4 minutes between sets.

NOTES: If you mess up at all during any of the 5-minute sets you must restart that set with no rest. This doesn't mean that you have to restart the entire workout, but just the set you're currently on.

The key to this workout is to develop a good pace that you can hold for 5 whole minutes. This workout isn't really too bad if you get it on the first try, but if you continue to make mistakes it will prove to be very difficult.

(2) 8 sets of the following:

- 40 double unders
- 15 push-ups
- 20 mountain climbers
- 10 burpees

*Rest 15 seconds between exercises and 2 minutes between sets.

(3) Complete the following as fast as possible:

- 3:00 double unders
- 6:00 freestyle skipping

- 10:00 plank
- 8:00 wall sit
- 2:00 burpees

*Rest as needed.

NOTES: The total exercise time for this workout is 28 minutes. This can be split up however you like by taking chunks out of each exercise time.

For example, you could do 30 seconds of double unders, 2:00 of freestyle skipping, 2:00 plank, 1:00 wall sit, etc. Just make sure you're keeping track of how long you're doing each exercise so you can ensure that you're not doing too much or too little. You can do the exercises in any order that you want.

(4) Perform 3 sets of the following:

- 1:00 jump rope
- 1:00 boxing jump rope
- 1:00 crossovers
- 1:00 ski skipping
- 1:00 jumping jack skipping
- 1:00 single leg skipping (right)
- 1:00 single leg skipping (left)
- 30 seconds double unders
- 30 seconds heel skipping

*Rest 30 seconds between exercises and 3 minutes between sets.

(5) 6 sets of 20 seconds on, 20 seconds off of the following exercises:

- Squat jumps
- Mountain climbers
- Double unders
- Push-ups
- Speed skipping
- Burpees

*Rest only 20 seconds between exercises and 1:30 between sets.

NOTES: This workout should be done at maximum intensity.

(6) 5 X 25 reps of the following exercises:

- Speed skaters
- Lunge walks
- Double unders
- Seal jacks
- Speed skipping
- Squat jumps

*Rest 30 seconds between exercises and 2 minutes between sets.

(7) Perform 4 sets of 30 seconds of each exercise:

- Heel skipping
- Double under crossovers

- Ski skipping
- Jumping jack skipping
- Boxing jump rope
- Double unders

*Rest 15 seconds between exercises and 2 minutes between sets.

THEN: perform jump rope for as long as you can until failure.

NOTES: The final part of the workout (max duration jump rope) isn't part of the main set and should only be done once the workout has been completed. Time yourself on this and try to see how long you can go for.

(8) You have 20 minutes to gain as many points as possible.

Each exercise corresponds to a point value; the harder the exercise, the more it's worth.

This workout is best done with a partner or a group so that you can compete to see who can gain the most points in the 20-minute time period.

- Speed skipping- 1 PT
- Seal jacks- 1 PT
- Mountain Climbers- 2 PTS
- Reverse crunches- 2 PTS
- Push-ups- 3 PTS
- Squat jumps- 3 PTS
- Double unders- 3 PTS

- Double under crossovers- 4 PTS
- Burpees- 4 PTS

*Rest as needed, but remember you need to get as many points as possible so rest responsibly!

NOTES: Try to ensure that even when you're resting, you're gathering some points by doing seal jacks or speed skipping.

(9) Perform 1 set of the following:

- 60 double unders, 60 seal jacks
- 50 double unders, 50 jumping jacks
- 40 double unders, 40 reverse crunches
- 30 double unders, 30 mountain climbers
- 20 double unders, 20 push-ups
- 10 double unders, 10 burpees
- 10 double unders, 10 burpees
- 20 double unders, 20 push-ups
- 30 double unders, 30 mountain climbers
- 40 double unders, 40 reverse crunches
- 50 double unders, 50 jumping jacks
- 60 double unders, 60 seal jacks

*Rest 30 seconds between every exercise and 2 minutes after reaching the halfway mark (upon completing the first set of 10 double unders and 10 burpees).

NOTES: This workout obviously requires a ton of double unders so make sure you're well warmed up!

(10) In 15 minutes, complete as many sets as possible of the following sequence:

- 20 speed skipping
- 10 double unders
- 5 burpees
- 10 lunge walks
- 5 squat jumps

*Rest when needed.

Once again, thank you for reading this book, and I hope you're getting a lot of valuable information. I would greatly appreciate it if you could take 30 seconds to leave me a review for this book on Amazon.com.

Enjoying this book?

Check out my other best sellers!

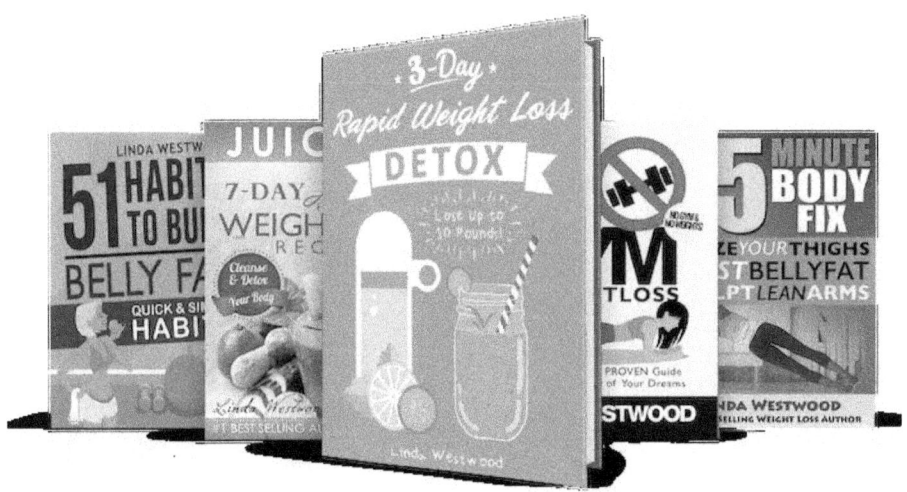

Get your next book on sale here:

TopFitnessAdvice.com/go/books

Chapter 5

Morning Habits

Habit 1: Wakeup Call

BUZZZZZZZZZZZZZZZZZZ!

Your alarm clock goes off. You're exhausted because you had a long day at work yesterday, but today is going to be different. Today is the first day you are going to practice the 30 ultimate habits that will revolutionize your life. So as soon as you hear that alarm clock go off, I want you to jump out of bed immediately.

Do not laze around trying to squeeze out a few extra minutes of sleep; it won't do you any good. In fact, if you don't get yourself up immediately and you spend 10- 15 minutes catching some last-minute sporadic sleep, it is going to make you more tired during the first half of your day.

Once you hear that alarm it's time to cut your losses and accept the fact that you now have to face reality. The morning is a difficult but crucial time for a lot of people.

If you have a rough morning, the rest of the day is sure to follow a similar pattern. But if you can manage to have a productive morning, the rest of the day will certainly be a productive one. So, do not press that snooze button, just shut that alarm off and jump directly out of bed.

If you need to do any thinking about the day ahead do it while standing or on your walk to the bathroom. This is going to sound painful, but I recommend waking up 20-30 minutes earlier than you normally do

Habit 2: Drink Up

Now that you're up and awake, it's time to hydrate yourself as soon as possible, head into the kitchen and pour yourself a tall glass of fresh water. Cut up a lemon and squeeze a piece into your water then drop it in. Put the remainder of the lemon in a zip lock bag and stash it in the fridge for the next few mornings.

Take a minute or two to drink this water and then poor yourself another glass to carry with you for the rest of the morning. Or you could just get yourself a big shaker bottle (BPA free) and fill that up from the get-go.

Drinking lemon infused water is a fantastic thing to do any time of day, especially in the morning. Lemon water is a great antibacterial cleanser because it helps control unhealthy viruses and bacteria in your body.

Lemon water will also reduce your levels of uric acid, which can lead to joint pain, as well as help your digestive system prepare for its first and most important meal of the day. Hydration is such a simple thing that so many people lack.

Water is an amazing and vital resource that has become more and more unpopular due to things like coffee, tea, Gatorade, energy drinks, milk and juice. Water should be your priority fluid as it is one of the main building blocks of humanity, other liquids are peripheral.

Habit 3: Get Moving

So far you should be about 5 minutes into your day so it's time to get your body moving immediately. A quick morning exercise routine is a very important habit to form. By getting yourself moving early in the morning you are saying to your body,

"Hey, this is what's going to happen. We're going to do a quick workout so that we can become energized once the endorphins get released. Get used to all of this movement because we are going to be going at this pace for the rest of the day!"

Getting your blood flowing will wake you up better than any amount of coffee ever could. I am the only person in my friend group who has never drank coffee in my life, even throughout a 5-year university program littered with late night studying and sleep deprivation. This amazes a lot of my friends and they ask me how I survive without coffee.

Well, none of the people that ask me this question do a morning exercise routine, and that is the answer to their questions. I supplement the stimulating properties of caffeine with push-ups, burpees and squats. Here is the exercise set I normally do, depending on the amount of time I have on a given morning.

2 or 3 sets of: 5 burpees, 10 pushups, 15 squats.

Make sure you are hydrating during and after this quick workout is complete. You shouldn't be totally exhausted once these exercises are done, they are not meant to be strenuous. You just want to put in a good five or ten minutes of movement to get your heart rate up.

Habit 4: Loose Goose

Stretching time. Once you complete your quick workout, before you eat it is time to do a quick stretching session. Look online to find stretches for different body parts. I recommend stretching the following areas: Your legs, groin, lower back, chest, neck and triceps.

By stretching, you enable your body to become more loose and flexible. I recommend stretching after every workout, not extensively after a short workout like the one you just completed, but at least a little bit.

Using a foam roller is almost the equivalent of getting a decent massage. These rollers are great for the back, legs, glutes and hips. If your job requires you to sit for the entire day, then this habit is very important for you.

Being sedentary for too long decreases flexibility at a rapid rate. The loss of flexibility is a surefire way to feel less energetic and more sluggish throughout the day.

Habit 5: Super Smoothie

You must be starving by this point so let's calm that craving. You've heard the saying before that breakfast is the most important meal of the day, and it is.

You want the first foods that you deliver to your body to be nutritionally rich and packed full of foods that are conducive to giving you the energy that you deserve and need. Grab your blender and let's make a super smoothie.

Throw in 1 frozen banana, 5 dates, half a cup of frozen blueberries, a handful of kale and spinach, ground flax seed, chia seeds, coconut water, unsweetened vanilla almond milk, half an apple, a spoonful of natural peanut butter, a teaspoon of matcha powder and a tablespoon of cinnamon.

The possibilities of smoothies you can make are virtually infinite. The above is simply one of my favorites and I guarantee after you drink it you will feel fantastic.

The smoothie may not look appetizing in color but your body will thank you for drinking it, I promise. There are a ton of brain foods in this smoothie and there is no doubt your mind and body will feel sharp after drinking it.

Habit 6: Extra Eating

Some mornings my smoothie is not enough to hold me over, so I need to eat something else. If you feel the same way, I recommend some of the following:

- A couple scrambled eggs

- A banana with some natural peanut butter spread on it

- An avocado spread on crackers

- A bowl of quinoa with cinnamon, pecans and almond milk added in

- Whole grain toast with coconut oil spread on it

- A plate of greasy nachos (just kidding, I'm just making sure you're still paying attention).

- A bowl of steel cut oats with cinnamon and almond milk

Habit 7: Vitamin Fix

With breakfast, I like to take 500mg of vitamin C, 1000 IU of vitamin D, one Jamieson Vita-vim multivitamin, 1200mg of fish oil, and 1200 mcg of vitamin B12. Speak to a doctor or nutritionist before taking any of these supplements, but I do not foresee it being an issue. I like to ensure that my body gets all of its necessary nutrients before heading off to tackle my day.

I find vitamin C significantly boosts my immune system and the only two times I have been sick in the past 5 years is when I neglected to take my vitamin C. Vitamin D is great because it provides you with the nutrients normally delivered to your body via the sun.

I mostly take vitamin D during the cold Canadian winters. Multivitamins provide you with a myriad of different supplements (depending on the brand), all of which are fantastic for your body.

Fish oils provide your body with essential omega 3 fatty acids, which help out with joint lubrication and brain function. Vitamin B12 helps with normal brain and nervous system function.

Habit 8: Ice, Ice Baby

The short workout is complete, you're well fed and it is time to shower. Take the idea of a nice long, relaxing shower and throw it out the window. This shower is going to make our minds alert, our bodies fit and have us feeling completely replenished.

Get into the shower, just as you normally would. Do your usual routine and then prepare for something drastically different. Step outside of the warm water and turn the water to as cold as you can bear. Step back into the stream and let the ice-cold water run down the back of your neck.

This will be uncomfortable and you will likely jump around a bit. This is a mental challenge more so than a physical one, do not give in to your urge to jump out of the shower, or turn the water warm.

Let the cold water hit every part of your body, control your breathing and try not to let yourself start sucking an excessive amount of oxygen. You will feel short of breath, but you need to keep telling yourself that everything will be ok.

Your body's natural reaction to freezing water is panic, because obviously if you are exposed to freezing cold water for too long, your body will start shutting down. Don't worry; you only need to stay under the water for three to five minutes (try for five!).

Once your watch tells you five minutes are up, you can turn the water warm again for ten seconds in order to regulate your body temperature, and then hop out of the shower. Who needs coffee right? If the workout didn't wake you up, this will wake you up like a kick to the teeth.

Cold showering is not an easy thing to do, but the benefits of them are miraculous. Your mind will be extremely alert, your hair and skin will feel fresher than ever, your circulation will be top notch, your muscles will feel rejuvenated, since you literally just shocked your body and convinced it that it might be dying soon, your instinctual priority list has shifted completely.

Survival instincts tend to flush out any peripheral thoughts that are not vital to that particular moment, meaning that you will feel less stressed and more relaxed.

Hopefully I have given you enough reasons to subject your body to the pains and chills of cold showering. Please don't knock it until you try it, seriously, it works wonders.

Habit 9: Self-Motivation

Once you step outside that shower and dry off, after you brush those fangs and check yourself out in the mirror, I want you to stare deeply at your reflection.

Take a moment to appreciate the opportunity you have been given to live out your current day. Reflect on the fact that just you being here, alive on this planet, is the ultimate lottery victory, with odds so incomprehensibly slim, that your mind can't even begin to fathom them. One hiccup in the past, one wrong decision by your mother or father, or their mother or father, or their mother or father and you would cease to exist.

The air we breathe right down to the earth we stand on is a complete miracle. Are you going to waste this miracle? Are you going to, even for one second, take this miracle for granted? No, you wouldn't even think about being complacent in this gift we call life.

You're going to go about your day with unprecedented zeal and energy. You're going to attack this day with a burning fury. Your body is a complex machine and if any of its vital parts decides to quit, consciousness as you know it will be gone forever.

A lot of people will tell you to live every day like it's your last, but not me. I know that my last day on earth would not be one that I'd be very proud of. It would probably consist of a lot of skydiving, riding motorcycles WAY too fast and just so, so, so much sex. I want you to live every day in gracious way.

Be appreciative of the things you have and do not dwell on things you don't. Attack every day with a passionate attitude and live every day like it's your very first day alive. Live it like you just sucked your first breath of fresh air after almost drowning in the ocean. Live it like you died and came back for a final chance at success.

Habit 10: Put It on Paper

Take out a piece of paper or your phone and make a checklist. This checklist will aid you in completing all of your daily tasks/goals. Checklists are a great way to hold yourself accountable, and they allow you to feel accomplished when you draw that beautiful check mark on the page.

By breaking your day down into a visible format, it allows your brain to better comprehend what you need to do and you will subconsciously begin planning out the steps you must take to in order accomplish everything on your list.

Normally, the difference between successful people and unsuccessful people is procrastination. By having a written list in front of your face, I find it becomes more difficult to procrastinate.

While you're at it you should also take the time to write down goals. These could be financial goals, career goals, relationship goals, fitness goals, or anything you want. Write weekly goals, monthly goals, yearly goals, 5 years goals and even ten-year goals.

Habit 11: Fill Up with An Extra Kick

Now it's time to head off to work, school, the gym or wherever you must go today. Before leaving you should fill up a large water bottle with ice water and a teaspoon of chia seeds.

If you have a transparent water bottle people might ask you if you are consuming frog eggs. These seeds are tasteless and you can drink them with ease. They will provide you with energy throughout the day by giving your body intermittent doses of omega 3 fatty acids, high quality protein and a ton of antioxidants.

There are very few calories in chia seeds, meaning they have a very high cost-benefit ratio when it comes to calorie intake. You get a lot without having to consume a ton.

Don't forget to share your thoughts on this book by leaving a review on Amazon.com. It takes just a few seconds.

Chapter 6

Afternoon Habits

Habit 12: Rock Your Body

Workout! You can do this wherever it fits into your schedule.

Right now, if you're saying to yourself "but I already worked out when I woke up," You did not.

What you did was a brief exercise set to get your blood pumping and ensure that your body was awake.

A real workout is a lot more extensive and it will require a bit more time.

I will provide some brief examples of workouts that you could do during the day, most of which do not require a gym, or any kind of equipment for that matter.

    A. 15-minute walk/ run.
       3x10 reps of:
       Pushups*, bodyweight squats, sit ups.

    B. 3 sets of 1 minute of each exercise:
       jumping jacks, mountain climbers, burpees, flexed arm hang, reverse crunches, squats (rest 3 minutes between sets).

C. 1 x 1 minute, 1 minute off, 1 minute on of each exercise: squat jumps, plank, burpees, flutter kicks, kettle bell swings.

D. 6 x 1 minute sprint, 1 minute walk (running).

E. 30-minute jog, every 5 minutes perform 3 burpees and 15 squats (stop the time when you do these exercises then resume jogging).

Try your best to make your workouts fun! Make sure you are constantly changing your exercise routine up because your body adapts very fast and you must keep it guessing. Track your progress and keep a workout journal so you can see how far you've come.

Hold yourself accountable to your workout schedule with an incentive system. If you miss a workout, then add an extra set to your next workout, or add another mile onto your next run.

Alternatively, if you are consistently following your workout schedule, make sure you give yourself relaxing rest days and allow yourself to eat some 'cheat foods' every now and again.

Habit 13: Don't Waste Your Downtime

Listen to good information, not repetitive music. If you have a long commute to work or wherever your day takes you, listen to audio books or podcasts. Instead of listening to "Shake It Off" for the 6th time in a row, give Taylor Swift a rest and listen to something educational and inspiring.

There are tons of great audio books out there and even more podcasts. You can find a podcast on any topic you want, subscribe for free on iTunes and listen at your own leisure. The last job I worked was at a grocery store and the only thing that kept me sane was listening to motivational podcasts, namely, The Joe Rogan Experience, which I highly recommend to everybody.

Habit 14: Positivity

Realize that your thoughts truly do impact your reality. I'm not promoting the book "The Secret," in fact one of my favorite quotes about this book was said by comedian Dave Chappelle:

"This book tells people that the secret to life is positive imagery, try flying to Africa and telling those starving children that shit. All you have to do is visualize some roast beef, taters and gravy. The problem is you have a bad attitude about starving to death."

Obviously, there is nothing funny about children starving in Africa, but Chappelle uses his comedic wit to make a really good point here. You cannot, as "The Secret" teaches, will things into existence with positive thinking and imagery.

Thoughts do impact reality a lot, but not to the extent that this book would lead you to believe - and yes, I have read this book cover-to-cover. You need to keep a positive mindset no matter what. Negative thinking only leads to more negative thinking, thus more negative results.

Positive thinking leads to positive outcomes and thus more positive results. Both mindsets are cyclical; the latter is just a lot more beneficial than the other.

Habit 15: S-T-O-P

I know the statement 'stay positive' is very broad but I believe the key to positive thinking is altering your internal dialogue. If you always have negative thoughts bouncing around in your head, it's time you change that. You must learn to talk to yourself in a positive manner. I know this sounds very corny and believe me, when I was first told to do this, I laughed.

But it really can make a massive difference in the way you conduct yourself and the way others see you. Some of the nicest people I know are also the most self-deprecating people I have ever met.

Sometimes it is necessary that you are critical of yourself, your actions or a decision you made, but it is not healthy to never give yourself positive feedback. I find women are especially bad at giving themselves the credit they deserve.

During the day, I want you to follow this simple acronym any time you are feeling down about something in your life.

S-T-O-P: Sit, Think, Objective, Positivity

Take a seat somewhere that you can be alone for a few minutes. Think about what's on your mind, or whatever is troubling you at that moment. Be objective and try to look at the issue or decision, free of bias, from a neutral third-party standpoint. Look at all of the positive aspects of whatever it is that is troubling you.

Habit 16: Live in the Now

"The now is here, the past is gone and the future will be nothing if the now is wrong." I made this quote up a few years ago when I was struggling financially. The message is that you must live in the now.

Dwelling on the past or future too much is completely pointless. Sometimes in life you are going to have to feel out of control, and that's fine. You must train yourself to not panic and to only worry about the things that you can control on that given day. The more in the now you can live, the happier you will be.

I am constantly trying to minimize the time frame that I concern myself with. You can start big and then keep shrinking your time frame like I did. Let me explain; I began by forcing myself to only worry about the week in front of me. I eventually shrunk that down to a few days and before I knew it I was down to one single day.

It felt great to only think about one day at a time and I noticed a jump in my productivity levels. I am currently working on cutting my time frame down to an hourly level, but that requires more practice.

Obviously, I am not telling you to completely ignore events that are coming up in your future, or to not learn from mistakes you have made in your past. All I'm saying is that once you gain the information you need from past or future events, it's time to let them go and not dwell on them. Do not beat a dead horse, let the past be the past and welcome the future when it comes.

Habit 17: Be Selfish Sometimes

Keep yourself motivated. This is certainly easier than it sounds, but by adopting the proper mind state, staying motivated can be very easy.

> *"I don't have to prove anything to anyone, I only have to follow my heart and concentrate on what I want to say to the world. I run my world"*
> *-Beyonce*

Beyonce Knowles just might be the most motivated female on the planet. Did you know while she was acting on a movie once that she was so determined to play her role perfectly, that she forgot to eat for two days? This woman is a true inspiration and I don't know many people, male or female, that have anything negative to say about her.

Keeping yourself motivated on a daily basis can be tiresome but you must always keep your goals at the front of your mind. By always reminding yourself of your daily goals, it allows you to persevere through whatever obstacles you may face. This is why in the earlier habits I told you to write your goals down so that you could physically see them on the paper.

When it comes to completing your goals, being selfish is ok. Make sure you get your own stuff done before you start spreading yourself thin in an attempt to please others. It's like when you're on a plane and the announcement comes on that says,

> *"If the cabin pressure changes drastically, an oxygen mask will deploy from above your head. Please safely secure your own mask before helping others with theirs."*

They say this because if you try to help others before you help yourself you may pass out, then two people are in trouble instead of just one. You are better able to help others once you help yourself first, never forget that and do not feel that being selfish is always a bad thing.

> *"I attribute my success to this: I never gave or took any excuse."*
> -Florence Nightingale

Habit 18: Role Models

Surround yourself with motivated, inspirational and positive people. If you only have friends that put your dreams down, over-criticize you, or flake out on plans on a regular basis, then maybe it's time to get some new ones.

Many people will do virtual Facebook friend cleanses, whereby they remove people that they no longer have a need for, off of their friends list. Why don't more people do friend cleanses in real life?

I know tons of people that have that one friend from elementary school that constantly drags them down. Those friends who can just never seem to dig themselves out of a rut, and they constantly drag others into that rut with them. Just because you have been friends with someone for a long time, does not mean you have a forced life sentence of friendship to serve.

Removing stress from your life requires you to remove stressors. If you have people in your life that are stressors, you need to minimize the time you spend with them, so as to minimize your own stress levels.

This may seem like a daunting task and it's true that cutting ties with people is much more difficult in the technologically advanced age that we live in. Learning to tell people no is an important skill to develop and by saying no to being friends with negative people, you will better develop this vital skill.

Habit 19: Limiting Stress

If you're finding that you cannot remove particular stressful people from your life i.e., your boss, coworkers, family members etc. Then you must learn how to limit the amount of stress that they are putting upon you. One way to do this is to keep them content.

If somebody is frustrating you, you must learn to control your emotions. Take some deep breaths and let's go back to the S-T-O-P method. Ask yourself if you are being reasonable.

Take a minute to reflect on the particular person that is creating the problem for you. Think of one positive thing about the person. I know this sounds childish and silly but it allows you to calm your frustrations. Even the most annoying people on earth have positive aspects to their personalities, whether it is tenacity, boldness, dedication, zeal, enthusiasm, punctuality, or a sense of humor. Once you have identified something positive that they bring to the table you will be able view the situation with a more unbiased lens.

There will be times where people in your life act in totally evil and irrational ways. During these times, you will have to take a different course of action. If somebody starts yelling at me, or taking out his or her anger on me, I try to remain as calm as I can.

By remaining calm you force the other person to feel foolish and embarrassed. These feelings will cause them to reevaluate what they're doing and potentially back down from the confrontation.

Just think; fire (anger) is aggressive and sporadic, if you mix fire with fire you will only produce a larger flame. Water (passivity) is calm and soothing, if you mix water with fire you can put out a potential inferno.

Habit 20: Nap Time

Sometime during the day, if possible, take a twenty-minute nap. I know this won't suit everyone's lifestyle, but if you can fit it in, then you definitely should. Twenty minutes has been proven to be the optimal napping time.

If you nap for too long, you will feel even more sluggish than you did before. This is because your body thinks that it is bedtime, so it begins to enter a deeper level of sleep. Twenty minutes is just long enough to give you a good shot of energy during your day- and trust me it works very well.

Others who are considering purchasing this book would love to know what you think. If you could spare a few seconds, they would greatly appreciate reading an honest review from you. Simply visit the page on Amazon.com.

Chapter 7

Evening Habits

Habit 21: Walk it Off

Once you get home from your long day of doing whatever it is that you do, I advise you take a short walk to blow off some steam. You don't have to walk for too long, I'd say 10-15 minutes at minimum.

During this short walk, you should reflect on the day that you just had. Determine whether or not you have accomplished all of the goals that you set for the day.

If the day didn't go well, think about what you can do during the evening to make it better.

If the day went well, then momentum is on your side and you should have no problem having a productive evening. Walking in the evening is also a fantastic idea so that you can get some exercise before eating dinner.

Habit 22: Snack Time

Have a quick snack directly following your nap. By having a little snack now, you will reduce the amount you need to eat at dinner in order to feel full. Overeating is never a good thing and it's clearly no way to lose weight.

Make sure the snack is not significant, perhaps a cliff bar or a banana dipped in natural peanut butter. If you have too big of a snack, you will stretch your stomach out and at dinner you will eat like a beast. Trust me, I've done it.

Habit 23: Read a Book

Catch up on some reading. Reading is great, mind stimulating activity. It keeps your brain sharp and it is something that you should do every single day.

Let your mind wander off into the different realms of the books that you indulge in. Studies show that reading helps to reduce stress, by removing your thoughts from your life and focusing them upon the words on the page.

Habit 24: Kill the Distractions and Meditate

Turn your phone to airplane mode, shut off the television, walk away from the computer and begin to meditate in a quiet location. If you do not know how to meditate, you have infinite resources on the Internet- from YouTube to books and articles.

Meditating obviously helps to reduce stress if done properly. The goal is to let go of any thoughts, positive or negative. Let your mind enter a state of emptiness where there is no concern or emotion.

If you can get to this relaxed state you will get a massive body high once you finish meditating. I never understood meditation until I experienced the amazing natural high that is associated with it. Now I try to meditate at least once a day.

Habit 25: Healthy Eating

It's time for a delicious healthy dinner. Here are some healthy dinner selections that I like to eat often.

- A) Mango avocado salad. I use one mango and avocado, cut them up and add black beans, lettuce, jalapeños, quinoa, salsa and low-fat corn chips.

- B) Mini pita pizzas. Add some pesto to pita bread with tomatoes, red pepper, onions and cheese. Bake the pita by the oven by itself first, add everything else and then put it back in the oven until the cheese melts

- C) Spaghetti squash cooked in the oven. I like to add crushed tomatoes or a little bit of pesto.

Eating a healthy dinner is vital if you want to keep/get a good figure. It's amazing what a difference cutting unhealthy foods out of your diet can make in your life. When cooking anything in a pan I would advise that you use coconut oil instead of regular cooking oil.

Coconut oil is a truly amazing saturated fat and the health benefits of it seem to be limitless. Coconut oil is great for the skin and it can even help you lose weight if consumed in moderation. It is fairly dense and it will help to fill your stomach so that you don't need to fill it with unhealthy fats.

Habit 26: Lose the Bad Food

It's fine to eat some unhealthy food from time to time, let's be honest we all do it. But since a lot of us cannot control ourselves (myself included) it's best to keep unhealthy food out of our living environment all together. If it's not there you can't eat it and if all you've got is healthy foods, well you either eat that, or you starve.

Habit 27: Make a List

If you want to take some time off of your morning routine you could use your downtime in the evening to write your goal list for the following day. Writing goals in the morning may be stressful if you are on a time crunch.

If you have the time in the evening, I recommend writing your daily goals for the following day, so you can really put in the necessary thought that this activity deserves. As I stated earlier, the more you make your goals physically visible, the more productive and successful you will be.

Habit 28: No More Food

Do not eat ANYTHING after 9:00pm. Eating soon before bedtime results in unnecessary weight gain. This is an easy habit to get into, simply set an alarm on your phone for 9:00pm. Once that alarm goes off you can either grab one last quick snack, or you can stop eating for the remainder of the night.

Consuming food before you sleep means that you have excess calories that cannot be expended because you are motionless in bed. You need to make sure that the calories that in put in your body have the chance to get burned off before you sleep.

Habit 29: Daily Reflection and Stretch

It's almost time for bed but we've got a few more things to do yet. During your nighttime ritual of teeth brushing, face washing and all of that good stuff take a minute to reflect. Look at yourself in the mirror just as you did in the morning and smile. Hold that smile until it becomes awkward and give yourself credit for everything you got done.

Head into your bedroom, but before jumping into your comfortable bed, pause. Reach your hands up into the air as high as you can and get onto your tippy toes. Stretch your entire body out and hold this position for as long as you can.

After you can't hold the stretch any longer, I want you to perform 10 squats (try to keep your legs parallel and get your bum right down to the floor. Keep your arms directly in front of you). Perform this stretch/squat set three times for a total of 30 squats.

This brief exercise set will not only tone your bum a bit (if done every night), but it will also help you sleep better. By slightly exerting your body before bed you will allow for better digestion of your dinner and a small fatigue of your muscles will help you drift off to sleep very quickly.

Habit 30: Set a Decent Bedtime

Make sure you are getting to bed at a decent time.

Aim to get 6-8 hours of sleep every night. If you don't get yourself into a consistent sleeping pattern, then you will never be at your best. If for some reason, you have to cut your sleep time down, try to add an extra 20-minute nap the following day, so that you can re-energize.

Sleep is obviously vital for both mental and physical health, so ensure that you get proper amount or else you will be feeling stressed and fatigued the following day.

I hope you have learned something from this book so far and would greatly appreciate it if you could leave an honest review on Amazon.com.

Chapter 8

Tracking Your Progress

One area that has really helped me stay focused while creating my healthy lifestyle has been the tracking and measuring side of exercising. I'm not a huge numbers person, I don't even really keep track of my Google analytics for my website, but what I have learned is that if I don't track and measure my weight loss and subsequent maintenance program, then I find it far easier to "fall off the wagon".

One of the easiest ways to track your progress is to simply jot down your measurements. I don't actually weigh myself on scales; instead I take the measurements of my arms, waist, hips, legs and chest area. This tells me how many inches I've lost, which relates to body fat.

This is a far better indicator of weight-loss progress than what you see on the scales, because muscle is heavier than fat, so when you're just starting out, your fat is being turned to muscle... it can take a little longer to reflect weight loss on scales.

So, do yourself a favor and measure your body fat instead. It's rewarding to see inches falling off week after week rather than checking the scales and seeing no change at all.

Here are some of the apps you can use to track and measure your progress:

1. **Simplenote App** - if you want to "write" your details down, this is a simplistic app that takes away all the fuss. I use this app to jot down what I did during my exercise session rather than taking down my measurements.

2. **Tracker** - Fitness and Nutrition Tracking - this app is great to not only track your workouts and weight/body fat, but you can also track your nutrition, which is great if you're struggling to stay on top of the food you're eating.

3. **Weight Loss Tracker** - this will purely track your weight and body fat, based on the information you provide it. It's a nice, simple app for anyone that is looking to just track their weight loss or keep an eye on their weight for maintenance purposes. iPhone and Android compatible.

4. **Fitlist** - Workout & Fitness Tracker - this is my favorite. You can enter in your own workouts and track your progress over time. This is what I'm currently using in conjunction with my spreadsheet. iPhone and Android compatible.

I can't reiterate enough how important it is to keep track of your weight loss/maintenance progress. Tracking and measuring are important to the success of your weight loss and it will also drive your maintenance program.

If you struggle with doing something like this, then definitely use one of the suggested apps, preferably Fitlist, Honestly, if I wasn't tracking my weight, I wouldn't be able to gauge my progress and I also wouldn't be able to monitor and make sure I am maintaining it.

I know that I spend most of my time during the day sitting, so I need to exercise to ensure the longevity of this body I'm residing in. I don't believe you need a gym to achieve the body or healthiness you're looking for, and evidently, neither do you – or you wouldn't have read this far!

I acknowledge that some people need a gym to achieve a certain look, and kudos to them, they can spend all the time they want at the gym. Me, I'm going to continue finding and developing different ways to stay fit that fit in with my lifestyle and that I can do in under 30 minutes a day.

I know that I'm preaching to the converted here, but seriously, why does society really feel the need to make us all work out in a confined space and dress in a certain way? Beats me.

It's one of those profound (I'm kidding!) questions that will never be answered. But I hope that I've been able to show you just how you can fit exercise into your day without joining the gym or owning equipment.

I hope you also realize that you have no excuse not to work out because everything in this book shows you that 30 minutes is all you need.

Discover Scientifically-Proven "Shortcuts" & "Hacks" to Lose Weight FASTER (With Very Little Effort)

For this month only, you can get Linda's best-selling & most popular book absolutely free – *Weight Loss Secrets You NEED to Know*.

Get Your FREE Copy Here:
TopFitnessAdvice.com/Bonus

Discover scientifically-proven tips to help you lose weight faster and easier than ever before. With this book, readers were able to improve their weight loss results and fitness levels. So, it's highly recommended that you get this book, especially while it's free!

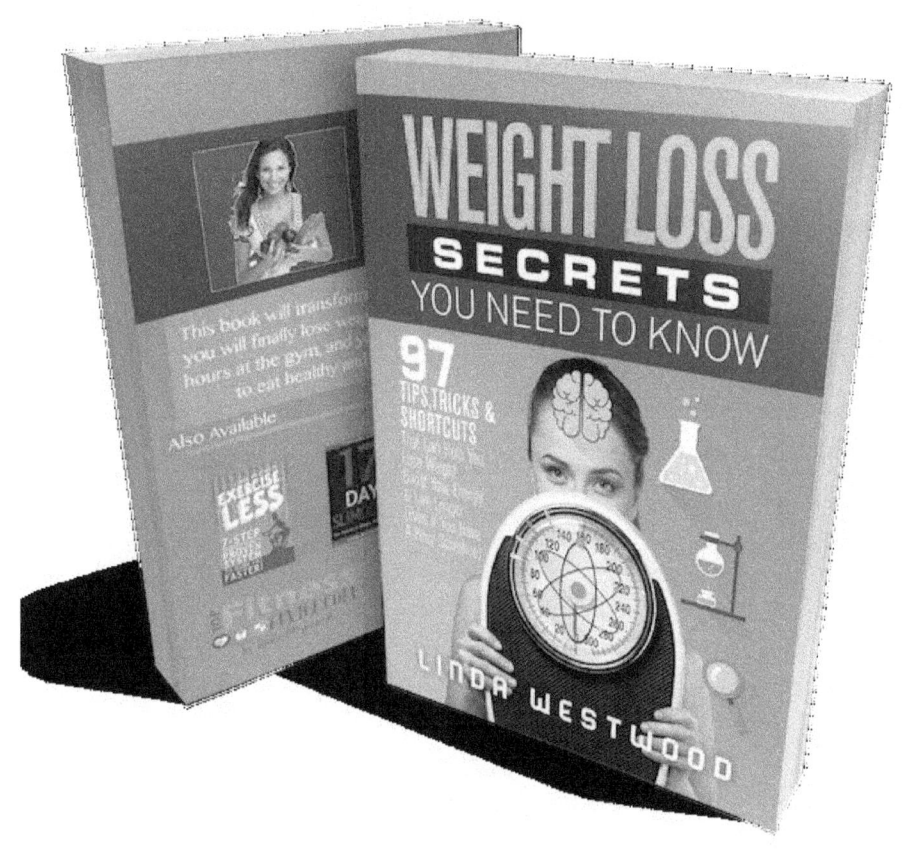

Get Your FREE Copy Here:
TopFitnessAdvice.com/Bonus

Conclusion

Great work on the workout program!

In conclusion, this book is merely a representation of my own personal experiences and the guidelines I try to follow in order to become a more happy and productive person. Everything I said is exactly what I do because it works very well for me, but this is not to say that it will work for you.

Modern life seems to trick our minds into thinking that "this is the way I should behave, sleep eight hours, work eight hours, eat when I can, have sex when I can, try to raise a family and repeat.

This is the cycle that traps many people and before they know it they are unhappy with their lives, likely due to the fact that they are unhappy with themselves. Just because our species has evolved in exponential ways over a brief period of time, doesn't mean we can forget our roots and genetics.

Our species conquered due to our rapid evolution of intelligence and fitness. Remember, it's survival of the fittest, not the mere existence of the complacent. We are at the top of the food chain because we have the physical abilities to act upon our ideas.

It's a well-known fact that human beings are the best long distance runners on planet earth. Yes, it's true that cheetahs could catch and eat us with ease. It would also not be wise to place a wager on a human at a horse race.

Humans could, however, run down both of these animals over a long distance until their hearts exploded, the reason? Sweat! Humans are able to sweat and when this sweat evaporates, our overall body temperature is cooled.

Many people hate sweating but I embrace this vital trait. Sweat lets me know that I'm exerting myself in an effective way and burning calories. Imagine if primitive humans behaved in the ways that the average person behaves today.

Lying around in caves, entertaining themselves with futile activities. We would have never made it out of that era and likely gone extinct if that was the case. The reason that didn't happen was all due to a lack of choice.

There were no T.V.'s, cell phones, iPods or things like that; there were only the priorities of food, shelter, water and reproduction. If you weren't mentally and physically fit enough you would perish, period.

Choice has quickly become societies enemy and has forever altered our priorities. Distractions have become so normalized that people forget what's important. It should be abundantly clear that we are not genetically designed to be sedentary all day.

Your body doesn't release endorphins if you beat a video game or finish a season of Breaking Bad. Endorphins are released under moments of stress, pain (like repeated exercise), and extreme pleasure. I think of Endorphins as a natural reward for doing something that will increase your chances of survival.

If sex didn't feel so damn good I guarantee we would have a less populated planet.

If you don't make time for physical activity in your life, you either will or currently are feeling the consequences. I think that if you trap and suppress your physical needs, your body has a tendency to "short circuit" and fulfill this physical need in other ways, such as violence or forced drama in your life.

I wish I could do an experiment on every single person on earth who suffers from depression, or who is just generally unhappy. I bet a large majority of these people do not exercise and I bet that if they did a lot of them would throw their prescriptions out the window.

I'm not trying to discount mental illness in any way. There are a lot of people who desperately need medication in order to function, due to major chemical imbalances in their brains. My point is that in some cases, people's feelings of emotional imbalance could be fixed or ameliorated through greater fitness levels.

Let's stop lying to ourselves, I mean who doesn't want to look into a mirror and say, "damn, I look great and all my hard work is paying off"? That's an awesome thing to desire and I think we all should.

Break your monotonous cycle and make room for your own fitness. Not only will you look better, but I guarantee you will feel more mentally and physically balanced as well.

If I have a difficult decision to make in my life, if I'm frustrated about something or if I just need some moving meditation, I go for a run or a swim and it helps immensely. I think there's something hypnotic about continuous movement. The ability to feel control over your entire body allows you to transfer this feeling of control to issues in your life.

This book will hopefully serve as your brief, yet difficult guide to a greater level of general fitness. Allow me to reiterate: Fitness is not a simple thing to achieve or maintain and anybody who tells you otherwise is lying to you, likely to make a quick buck off of you.

Fitness must be achieved, maintained and constantly improved upon. It is a lifestyle choice that will make you a happier person. You only have one body, so why not make it the best physical specimen that you possibly can.

Final Words

I would like to thank you for purchasing my book and I hope I have been able to help you and educate you on something new.

If you have enjoyed this book and would like to share your positive thoughts, could you please take 30 seconds of your time to go back and give me a review on my Amazon book page.

I greatly appreciate seeing these reviews because it helps me share my hard work.

You can leave me a review on Amazon.com.

Again, thank you and I wish you all the best!

Enjoying this book?

Check out my other best sellers!

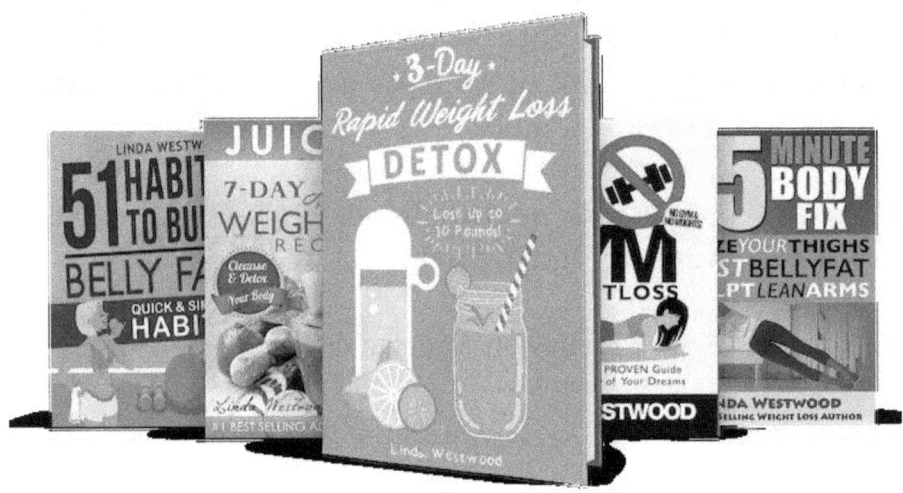

Get your next book on sale here:

TopFitnessAdvice.com/go/books

www.ingramcontent.com/pod-product-compliance
Lightning Source LLC
Chambersburg PA
CBHW031202020426
42333CB00013B/769